FLOWER POWER

Redefining the Paradigm

of Patient Care

SUSAN C. DEWEY, R.R.T.

Susan C. Dewey

DEDICATION

This book is dedicated to my loving mother Marlene Dewey, who lost her life to caregiver indifference, and to my family, who made the decision to uphold her wishes and end her suffering. Her life of caring about others and making a difference inspired this book.

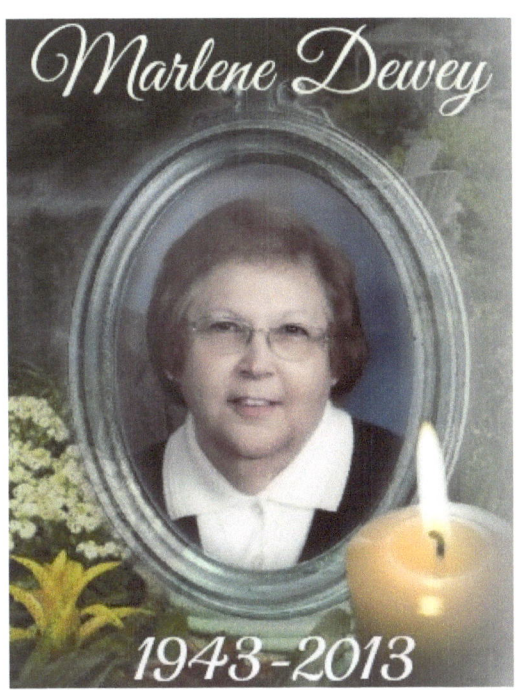

Also, to my family and friends for their support and encouragement while this project developed from my crazy idea into my first experience as an author. Throughout this journey of learning how to live my passion, I met and learned from many inspiring individuals, who urged me to believe in that passion and follow my dreams. I thank and also dedicate this to every one of you.

This book was written for those who work in our healthcare systems and facilities; those who wish they could speak up but are intimidated to do so, Healthcare staff and administrators who believe in doing the right thing and doing fulfilling work, administrators and CEO's who throw their hands up, at the seeming impossibility of working with stringent legislation and regulations.

This book is also for every patient entrusting us with his or her care. Those patients who come from any walk of life, those that come to us for our help in a vulnerable time. They expect to be cared for without judgment, with dignity, respect and humanity. They come to us to be treated like human beings, expecting us to care for their minds, bodies, and spirits. They do not come to be treated with indifference. Rich or poor, homeless and unkempt or living in mansions, well-educated or not, surrounded by family or alone, struggling or thriving, democrat or republican, man or woman, black or white, foreign or American, we are all spiritual beings having a human experience.

ACKNOWLEDGEMENTS

I would like to thank:

My mother, Marlene, for the inspiration to follow my passion; my family -James Dewey, Lisa Ball, Mike Dewey, Daniel Dewey, Jim & Jessie Dewey, Marcus Wekenmann, Bridgette and Sierra Bickel, for seeing my passion and believing in me. Thank you.

To the countless friends and acquaintances I have made along this adventure who supported and motivated me, including: Amber Warren McCartney, Jenifer Nemeth, Jen Paulus, Amber Moon, Jim Livesay, Kendra Miller, Doug S., Delayne H. Thank you.

Susan C. Dewey

CONTENTS

Susan C. Dewey

INTRODUCTION

What if today you felt fulfilled by your work? Today you felt your work was rewarding because you delivered care to patients with kindness and compassion no matter who they were, or their circumstances. Today you were able to do the work your patients appreciate; work that felt fulfilling and right. It would be an unusual day because this is not how our day usually goes. This is a rare chance to be human, and care. It would go something like this:

Today you refilled a glass of ice water for a patient. You helped a nurse boost your patient up in bed. You used a wet cloth to wipe a patient's crusted eyes and sweaty face. You found a patient in a wheelchair too tired to continue, and gave them a push back to their room. You found a warm blanket for a cold patient and adjusted the thermostat. You escorted a lost, confused patient back to their room. You held the hand of, and comforted a family member stricken with grief by the news that their loved one may not survive. You visited a patient you had a week ago, to see how they were doing and be a friendly face. You helped a nurse save time when you added humidity to your patient's oxygen. While a patient received her treatment, you helped her with the snaps on her gown so she felt more comfortable. You listened as a patient shared their story of ministry and giving back to her community. You helped a nurse who was having trouble with oxygen equipment and a stubborn pulse oximeter. A patient care assistant was busy with a complicated situation in another room, so you helped a patient eat lunch.

None of these things relate to medication or doctors orders. So, why do them? Do them because they matter. They have a significant effect on our patients' perception of care; more so than any medications, tests, procedures, doctors orders or color coded scrub system. These brief, seemingly insignificant moments give patients the ability to see our human side. The compassionate side is often hidden under an unrealistic workload preventing us from delivering this type of care on a regular basis.

Too often our patients are written off by doctors and caregivers who don't understand the healing power compassion holds for our patients. The human touch is often a forgotten element in treating patients. If a patient thrashes around after sedation is withdrawn, the first inclination is to re-medicate them so they don't injure themselves. Do we ever stop for a moment to hold the hand of those patients and talked to them instead of reaching for more sedation? Why not? They are listening. How much power does the human spirit hold? How much can the human touch mean? Can a smile or hug make a difference? As human beings we have the ability to change another's life with the simple touch of our hands, or a smile on our face.

It only takes one single act of kindness to make a difference in many patient situations. If we did this more often, and were encouraged to do so by "the powers that be", how would that effect our patients perception of their care? What would it do to improve patient outcomes and satisfaction scores? What impact could doing fulfilling work have on our staff? Couldn't it be a win – win for everyone involved? How do we move forward out of the darkness of the current paradigm of patient care? Can we simply continue to keep doing what we've always done?

Yes, it's true. Our health care systems are plagued by layers of obstacles; challenge after challenge. It's a giant ball of twisted bureaucracy that is out of control. We may not be able to fix everything, but with a new approach and perspective isn't it possible we stand a chance at improving our workplaces and the work we do? Isn't it time we step back and reconsider a completely new approach to patient care? One which is structured in a fashion that compliments the bureaucratic changes that have been put in place rather than the failing cookie cutter fixes we've been trying.

"Death is not the enemy, gentlemen. If we're going to fight a disease, let's fight one of the most terrible diseases of all — indifference."

~ Patch Adams

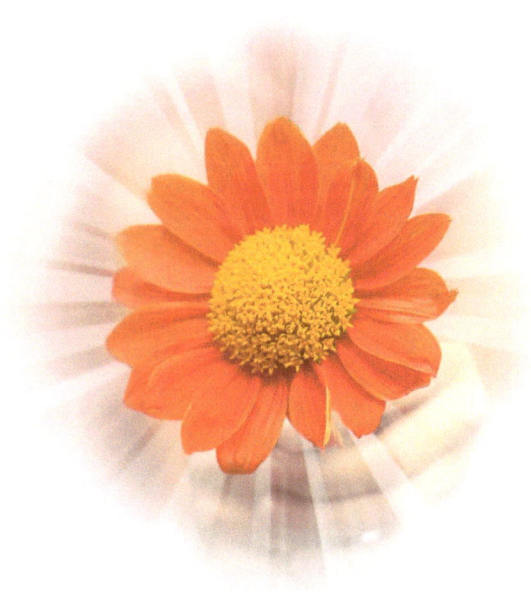

Susan C. Dewey

CHAPTER 1

THE TRAP OF INDIFFERENCE

The world we live in is plagued by indifference. Our schools, businesses, and even healthcare systems are failing under this poisonous reality. What is indifference? Merriam-Webster defines it as this:

> **indifference** – *Noun.* lack of interest in or concern about something: an indifferent attitude or feeling.

What's wrong about living with indifference, you ask? Well, let me ask you: What happens when we accept it and go along with it? People start doing whatever they want. People begin doing things that don't benefit anyone but themselves. People stop caring about what's right or wrong, and just start doing what's necessary for them to get by. How does that seem to be working out for us? In some fields, it might work out all right. Business might not be booming, but if you remain in business, it's okay. How does it feel to navigate this indifferent world that we live in? To me, it feels lonely. We don't and can't trust each other to do what's right. Doing the right thing and being indifferent do not go hand in hand.

In our healthcare system's indifference can mean life or death. It can mean the difference between a good outcome and a bad outcome. Many critical decisions have to be made by those whom we trust to care for us, those who are supposed to have our best interest in mind. In a world accepting of indifference, even trusted professionals won't care about what's in our, or your, best interest. It is the opposite of caring; both cannot work together. Every day that we continue to accept indifference as the norm, nothing will change.

I have worked in and traveled to many hospitals and seen the effect this indifference has on the care we deliver to our patients. I grew tired of accepting it to be my norm, or the standard to which I wish to be judged.

When I began my career as a Registered Respiratory Therapist, I was focused on applying what I learned in school and improving my skills. I thought I would be helping people and making a difference. Instead, I found a world full of negativity, apathy to patients, and conformance to the idea that we can't make a difference, so we'll just keep doing what we've always done: *Nothing*. When I joined this voiceless society and dove into my career, I found things to be very different from my expectation. As I have traveled to numerous other hospitals, I have borne witness to many things that I believe should have been fixed, improved, or changed in some way to make our patients' care and overall well-being better.

You see, to me it makes sense to heal the mind and spirit in addition to the bodies of our patients. This requires our treating them with dignity, respect, and compassion.

One of the first seemingly harmless incidents that comes to mind is the day I entered a patient's room to find my patient falling out of bed—crying, calling for help, and holding desperately onto the bed sheets to keep from sliding onto the floor. As I entered the room, I called for help to another caregiver outside the room, who entered and remarked, "She can get up on her own, she just doesn't want to. She has a walker." The caregiver then promptly turned around and left the room.

She was right; there was a walker, on the *other side* of the room. I could have gone to get her walker and brought it over, but I knew I had to help her without the walker because she had clearly already lost every ounce of dignity she had. She felt helpless, and if I let go, she was going to be on the floor. So, with her firm grasp on the bed linens, I gave her a boost and helped my crying patient up into bed and began her nebulizer treatment while I tucked her in and calmed her down. She didn't want me to leave. With a look of fear on her face she asked, "Will you be back?" I assured her that I'd be back and continued on my day. When I returned for the next round of treatments, the patient was sitting in her chair with her walker close at hand, smiling from ear to ear, and said, "I'm so glad you came back! Will you be here tomorrow?" I felt like I did something that mattered. It felt good to see her so happy. I immediately picked up on a sense of trust she now had in me. If our patients feel that they can count on us and trust us, their perception of us must be pretty good. Right? How does it feel for us as the caregiver? It feels fulfilling. Our patients do not want to lose their dignity, or feel helpless. It's up to us to decide when enough is enough and to just help them.

One morning at the beginning of my shift, I received a call from a nurse, asking me to take a patient off BiPAP and to put her on a high-flow nasal cannula so she could eat breakfast. BiPAP is a type of device commonly used when a patient either can't maintain good oxygenation or is not breathing efficiently enough to keep CO_2 levels from building up in their blood.

When I arrived to the bedside of a visibly frail, weakened woman, I removed her BiPAP and placed her on a nasal cannula. I informed her nurse, who happened to be in the doorway, and her only statement was, "Well, I hope she can feed herself, because I don't have time to deal with her!" I tried to help the patient with breakfast, but now she was not only frail, but emotionally distraught, and refused to eat. I was used to this type of thing; it happened day in and day out. I felt helpless. This nurse was overloaded with patients and work to do. I knew she didn't mean it that harshly, but what is one to do?

There are days like this. We all get sucked into the trap of indifference. Why? I'm not sure. Maybe sometimes it's just easier to focus on getting the work done so that no one has to ruin our day by mentioning productivity. Some days it just feels like the cards are stacked against us. Sometimes it might just be because we don't want to hear the "It's not my job," or "I don't care, I don't have time for that" comments. If we close ourselves off to caring on some days, we just survive and feel less tattered at the end of the day. In reality, what happens at the end of a day when you've fallen into the trap of indifference is that you leave work and go home feeling like you just didn't do a good enough job. It's never easy, whether focusing on caring in an environment that doesn't support it, or going with the flow of indifference. If you're someone who believes in caring about people, it just feels terrible. All the more reason to build an environment and team that supports our drive and mission to make a difference in our patients' lives. Going with the flow should mean falling into a pattern of caring and going the extra mile for our patients, but we don't. Why?

If you stand in the halls of your facility and look around at your staff, what do you see? Smiling faces? In most facilities, such as where I've worked, you rarely see this. We don't even smile at each other. We don't look or act like a team. How would any patient ever get a sense that we're on the same team? They wouldn't, and don't. We're all so separated by our indifference that instead of helping each other, we ignore and complain about each other. One would think that if we all had a common goal—to take care of our patients—we would work together, right? We don't have a common goal anymore. Some of us are just trying to survive the day. Some of us are trying to focus on getting the work done and focus our productivity where it needs to be, and a few of us are able to remain focused on actually caring for our patients. Indifference is the product of mismanagement and patient overload. It is an important factor, one of the most important when addressing patient care and our *ability* to care. I have worked on patient floors aside nurses who are assigned 6-8 patients. 1 nurse to care for 6-8 patients for 12 hours. The problem has prompted National Nurses United (www.nationalnursesunited.org) to petition for legislation mandating change in the nurse to patient ratios. Higher ratios are associated with more patient deaths, complications, and medical errors — "State Mandated Nurse Staffing Levels Alleviate Workloads, Leading to Lower Patient Mortality and Higher Nurse Satisfaction," Agency of Health Research and Quality, AHRQ Healthcare Innovations Exchange, Sept. 26, 2012. Proposed ratios have benefits for both patients and nurses. The California Nurses Association's historic first in the nation Safe Staffing RN Ratios law took nearly 13 years to win and has been in effect since January 2004 despite continued efforts of the hospital industry and then Governor Schwarzenegger to have it overturned or otherwise weakened.

We have reached the point of patient ratios that are dangerous to the patient and our staff. Whether we are discussing nursing, respiratory therapy, CNA, phlebotomy, radiology, or transport; it reaches a point where it endangers every one of us. Add to the current ratios the fact that facilities are considering significantly reducing respiratory therapy staff and giving the majority of our duties to nurses already managing dangerous workloads.

But who even notices? No one. No one, that's, except our patients and visitors. It has become a game of survival — everyone worried about themselves and their work. What their job is and isn't. Cohesive teams work together for the good of an outcome. In healthcare, that outcome is our patients' healing. Working as a team requires trust and respect, which many teams lack. When we work all day watching our backs and covering our butts, it's hard to walk around smiling. The ironic part of this is that smiling is an automatic stress and anxiety reliever. It seems we would have a much better day if we could just crack a smile once in a while. Our administrators create these great engagement programs, but never follow up to see if they're working, and if they're not, to see why they're failing. They rarely see what's going on in the daily environment of their staff.

Indifference separates and divides us all. It will cause us to fail every step of the way if it's not remedied.

Susan C. Dewey

"The best way to find yourself is to lose yourself in the service of others."

~Mahatma Gandhi

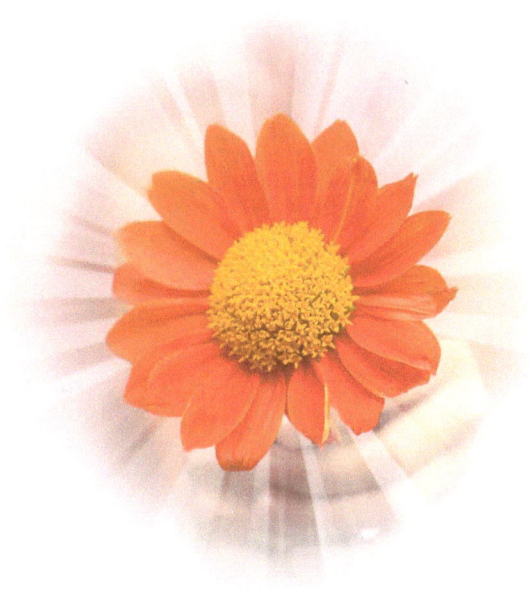

Susan C. Dewey

Chapter Two

CARING IS EVERYONE'S JOB

One morning, I came upon a patient whose care had been repeatedly neglected. My patient had a tracheotomy and was on a ventilator. This patient was awake and alert, sitting in a chair on CPAP (a mode on the ventilator that lets the patient breathe on their own with a little help) ready to be weaned off the ventilator. Since it was early in the morning, it was dark in the patient's room, and as a previous night shift veteran, for the patient's comfort, I don't usually turn bright lights on. I had enough light at the time, or so I thought.

As I began to remove the ventilator tubing from the tracheotomy, I noticed some things that didn't look quite right — things looked concerning and required me to see better. I let the patient know and proceeded to turn on the big overhead light. What I discovered was unbelievable! There were gaping, infected, oozing wounds of 4-6 inches surrounding this tracheotomy. There were dried unknown formations, and a rubber band holding the ventilator tubing to the trach so it wouldn't pop off due to the oozing wounds and cause the ventilator to alarm. The rubber band was being eaten away by bacteria in the wounds in which it was lying. The patient's trach was still sutured after 5 weeks and it was clear from my experience that very little trach care had been done in those 5 weeks (in my judgment, probably not even once).

If it had, the ties would not be blackened and filthy, blackened as if they'd been a pair of white socks worn outdoors without shoes for three or four days.

I called the nursing supervisor into the patient's room and showed her the problem I had. The nursing supervisor became my second pair of hands. Now, you have to realize that to work on a patient's trach, we're right up in their personal space. Our patient understood we were trying to help her, and was very still and attentive. The nursing supervisor had paged the doctor to have the sutures removed, and we continued assessing the wounds and trach. We came upon a hard, black, crusty-looking thing among the wounds and oozing. The nurse assisted me in determining what exactly we were looking at. I asked her, "What do you think this is? I don't want to pull on it. I'm not sure if it's dried secretion, dried blood, dead tissue, or what, but it's in the way." She wasn't sure, either. The patient was a true gem, going through all this fully awake and alert, while remaining calm and cooperative. The nurse took a pair of scissors and ever-so-gently trimmed just the very, very edge of this unknown object. We made a very concerning discovery; it was the end of a 4-inch strip of rotting gauze that was wrapped around the underside of the trach and around the trach itself inside the stoma (inside the patient's neck) The

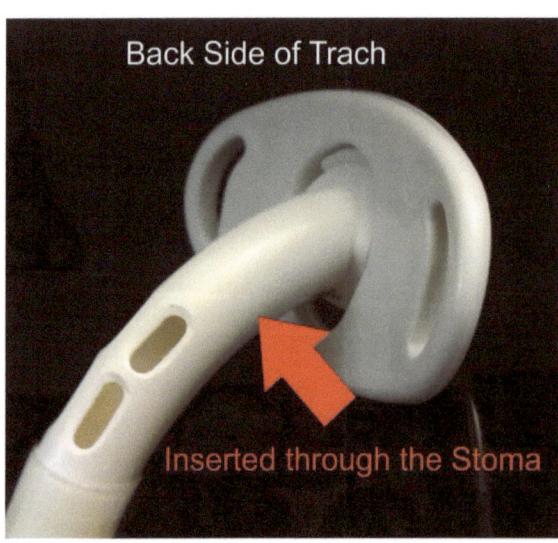

Back Side of Trach

Inserted through the Stoma

stoma is a hole in the neck that the trach passes through as it enters into the airway. That gauze appeared to be the most likely original source of infection. It was black, covered in pus and decaying tissue.

Similar to this, which was also found wrapped around a trach in a separate situation.

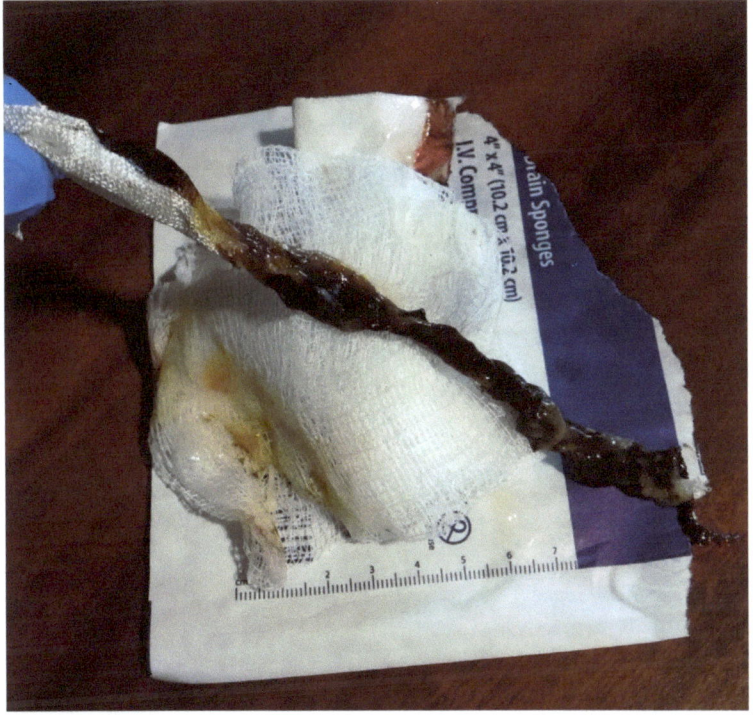

To say it smelled foul is an understatement. At this point I realized the gravity of this patient's condition, and clarified with the charge nurse what their policy was on removing sutures. In most hospitals, policy dictates that only a physician or surgeon can remove them. In this case, we had already been waiting 3 hours for a doctor to show up and remove them. I called my manager in an attempt to clarify the policy, and whether or not I could remove the sutures. He said, "Why are you doing trach care? That's the nurse's job." I tried to explain why it was so important, but he kept telling me to let the nurse handle it. He wasn't interested in what was going on with our patient, so I then hung up and I told the charge nurse to get me a suture removal kit. She adamantly refused, reminding me that I could be fired for removing the sutures because it's against policy. It didn't matter to me at this point, if I got fired for doing the right thing, then so be it. She convinced me to wait as she paged the doctor one last time.

There were gaping wounds full of infection from secretions and moisture, causing skin breakdown leading to wounds so deep, the plate of the trach (the oval-shaped piece pictured here) was recessed deep into the wounds. I just couldn't believe that no one had taken the time to care. It took 3½ hours and repeated calls to doctors to get the sutures removed to finish tending to this patient's trach care. When the doctor arrived, with about 5 medical students in tow, he removed the sutures and proceeded to leave room, indifferent to the condition of his patient.

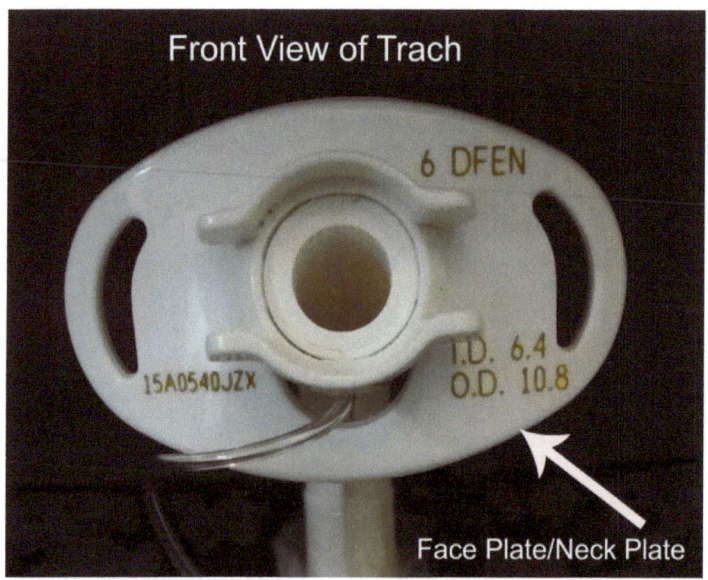

We completed trach care by cleaning the area as best we could, placing dressings over the wounds, and putting clean trach ties on. Then I called wound care to come evaluate and treat the wounds. She successfully saved me from losing my job, but more importantly, I believe, together, we saved this patient's life. At minimum, we prevented our patient's condition from declining and possibly having a poor outcome.

When I returned to my department that day, I inquired to our manager why we were using rubber bands to secure circuits to trachs, since, in my experience, I have never been aware of sterile rubber bands. Most rubber bands come from, oh, I don't know, our pockets, or the bottom of a dirty desk drawer. I was informed by my manager, "That's how we've always done it. It's how we will continue to do it." Then once again, he inquired, "Why are you wasting time doing trach care? That's not your job; it's the nurse's job." This is the first time I found my voice, I could not be quiet another second. "It's my job," I said. "I'm trained to do it, and it was the right thing to do because no one had taken time to do it or even cared that it hadn't been done." This was also the day I began being glared at by my peers. "Trouble" seemed to be my *new* label. There was one coworker who came to me and said, "You did a good job for that patient, but you know, no one really cares. They're just going to do what they've always done. No one can change that, not even you. I wish we could change things, but no one cares."

I appreciated the acknowledgement of doing the right thing, but was bothered by the belief that we can't make a difference and that no one cares. My patient cared that day, and thanked us over and over after enduring almost 4 hours of our efforts to care for them.

This is the current paradigm we work in. I'm trying to demonstrate the effects of how our current paradigm creates an environment that does not support caring for our patients, and fails to treat them as human beings. This industry we work in does not cater to caring for patients as human beings with dignity and respect. *Are* there "bad" nurses and therapists out there? Yes, there are. Until we support and create an environment that promotes fulfilling work, we will continue to staff those therapists, nurses, and heath care staff that would be better suited in other industries. You might be asking yourself, "Where does the blame lie?" The blame falls on each one of us who continues to support the indifference in our healthcare systems. It lies with those of us keeping quiet about the fact that we're not allowed to care.

Susan C. Dewey

"Our job is improving the quality of life,

not just delaying death."

~Patch Adams

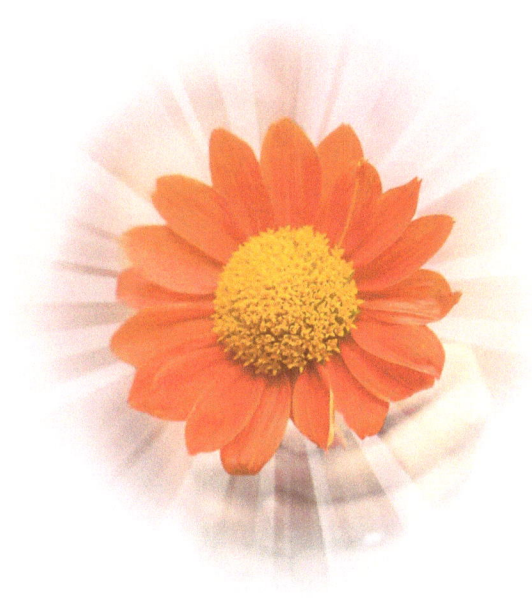

Susan C. Dewey

Chapter Three

THE PROMISE

Finding my voice has been a blessing and a curse, as speaking up is not encouraged; rather, it's discouraged. When you do speak up, you are disregarded, dismissed, and you start to honestly believe that no one cares, and that it's never going to change. What happened to doing the right thing? What happened to caring about our patients? Their well-being depends not only on medicine, but on their spirit, and how they feel emotionally. It also depends on us!

What happened that made me decide to speak up and try to make a difference? This book and mission are dedicated to my mother Marlene. Two years ago, my family and I gathered to say goodbye to her as she took her last breath and passed away. After her passing, I heard stories about her patient care and what she had to experience. I heard so many things that she had to go through that I see every day. I decided that I'm not going to be quiet anymore. That was *my mom*! That's someone else's mother, father, daughter, brother, aunt, or uncle. I can't change the world, but I'm not going to be quiet about something so important anymore.

When my mother was ill and not doing well, I traveled home a lot. I heard the story of her infections caused by caregiver indifference. I heard how a nurse told my father, "She needed to feed herself." Just like that frail, weakened patient on BiPAP I told you about earlier. My mother was so weak, she could not lift her arms, and she could barely speak. There was never any physical therapy done to strengthen her muscles, so please tell me, how in the world was she going to feed herself? She was passed along an indifferent team of caregivers until there was no hope for recovery. She had a severe infection from bed sores that were so deep they were down to her coccyx, or tailbone. She had another infection in her abdomen as deep as her pelvis. My mother was being eaten away by infection down to the bone. She was septic and malnourished. Her levels of albumin, a protein that helps keep fluid in our vessels, was so low in her blood, it was immeasurable—nearly undetectable. There was no return from that, and my family gathered as we withdrew life support and she passed on. After being quiet for so long about so many things, those same things happened to my own mother.

My mother was a special, unique woman. Don't we all believe our mothers to be? In her passing, I learned more about my mother than I did throughout my whole life with her. I learned things about myself as well. At her wake, or some call it a viewing, I recall noticing something I thought was unusual for the passing of a woman her age, 69 years young. I thought to myself, "Wow, look at all the people who came out in the freezing cold on icy roads to pay their respects and share their memories of my mother." It was early March in northern Indiana and in the low 30s. I realized that she touched ALL those people's lives, every one of them, so deeply they came out to say goodbye, and to let us know that she made a difference in their lives.

I stood in the back of that room in awe of her. I promised her that I would make a difference, too. I would make sure that I used this gift of caring about people that she gave me, the same one she possessed and used so eloquently, and use it as well as she did. I didn't know exactly how, but I made that promise with tears in my eyes and without hesitation. The way she touched people made their faces light up when sharing their stories and memories of her. It touched my heart and made me proud to be her daughter.

During conversations after the funeral, I heard those stories again. The stories of how she was failed by those who were trusted to care for her. It made me angry, and ashamed that I saw those things all the time and never spoke up. That was *my* mom those things had happened to, and no one ever needs to go through that, especially my own mom! I realized that I had to find my voice, for my mom, for my patients, and for my own conscience. Wasn't I just part of the problem if I never said anything and remained silent? Wasn't that, in a way, being indifferent like everyone else?

Susan C. Dewey

"You must not lose faith in humanity. Humanity is an ocean; if a few drops of the ocean are dirty, the ocean does not become dirty."

~Mahatma Gandhi

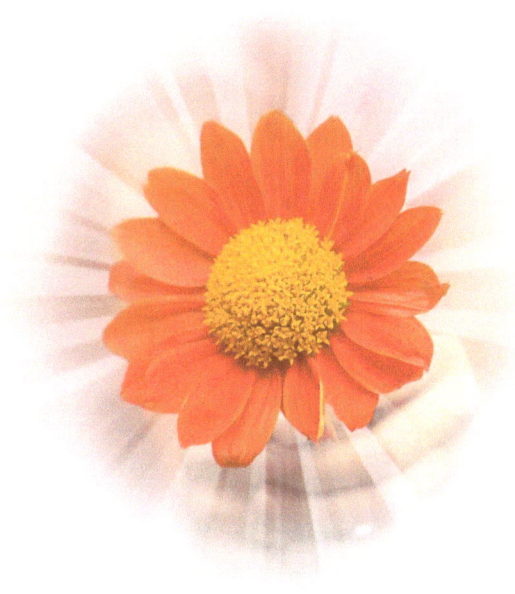

Susan C. Dewey

Chapter Four

THE PATIENT EXPERIENCE IS A HUMAN EXPERINCE

There was a patient who was constantly being missed when it came to their care. I saw this patient because they were a trach patient, as are many of my patients. I knew that, very often, trach care was not done unless I was assigned to their floor, so I regularly checked in on these patients. This particular day, I was doing trach care, cleaning everything, changing trach ties and equipment. I said that, at a minimum, the trach ties should be getting changed daily with trach care, just like they bathe this patient. My patient looked at me with tears forming in their eyes, filling up and about to spill over on their cheeks.

My patient said, "They won't give me a bath because they think I'm gross." They proceeded to tell me the last bath they had was four days ago, and the patient care techs on that day, and every bath day, comment out loud how gross it is. "They won't give me a bath, ma'am," my patient said, holding their head down in shame. I said, "You deserve to be bathed every day like every other patient. No one should be commenting on your condition or their opinion of it." It goes without saying that this patient's room did not smell delightful — there were gnats flying around it — but there was absolutely no reason for a single human being on this earth to be treated this way, especially in a hospital. This happens too often. We are so busy because of the way our facilities are run, that these patients are the last one's anyone want to deal with. They wait until someone gets around to them.

I remember the first time I encountered this patient. I discovered, as I often do, that trach care had not been done in quite some time. I looked into the EMR (electronic medical record) and saw that a nurse and respiratory therapist had charted that trach care had been done in the last 24 hours. The evidence I saw said otherwise. I called to the nurse, who was outside the room, and asked if she had completed trach care. She defensively stated she'd done it that morning. I invited her into the patient's room and asked her again, explaining that I couldn't understand why it looked as it did if trach care had been completed. I immediately sensed tension from the approach I used, but went on to suggest that if she'd go collect the supplies we needed, I would help her do the trach care on this patient. I watched her expression change from angry to thankful in a few short seconds.

I know that many seasoned nurses are not comfortable doing trach care, even other respiratory therapists struggle with it; so this nurse, who looked as if she were 15 years old—obviously a new nurse—was probably far from comfortable with the process. Educating and helping each other is a step in the right direction. Why are more of us not bridging these gaps? If we were, we wouldn't have situations like this. If there's a need for more training, then we should offer more training. The truth is, no one really ever speaks up, so nobody recognizes the need. Sometimes it just comes down to doing the right thing. If it means helping or training nurses and RTs or even physicians, then that's what we should be doing. I believe we need to take a good look at how to identify the problems, see what's really happening out there on our patient floors, and begin finding new solutions.

It's because of stories like these that I suggested for one hospital to institute trach rounds. I repeatedly saw that it wasn't being done, yet this affects the patient's outcome. I had previously worked at a hospital that put this idea into practice for the exact same reason. Trach care was not getting done and, when it was done, it was done in a substandard way. The implementation of the rounds was a huge success. It made therapists and nurses accountable and when further training was needed, it was clear.

At which point that training was done, even if it meant continuing to help another respiratory therapist or nurse complete trach care until they were comfortable doing it themselves.

One main reason trach care doesn't get done or done properly is because it's so intimidating. The first reason it's intimidating is because, if at any moment the patient coughs — which happens often during trach care — the trach could pop right out! Yikes! We don't want that to happen! That's bad! It's also because — God bless our nurses, who deal with all types of body functions and fluids — they're seriously grossed out by secretions of phlegm. They can handle everything else that I personally can't, which is why I think every nurse is an angel for what they do, but they're really uncomfortable around ooey-gooey trachs. When we teach each other how to overcome the intimidation and help them get used to it, it's a win-win for everyone. Needless to say, my suggestion was turned down by my manager. I went to infection control and pitched it again. Turned down. I went to the director of nursing, turned down. They actually told me it was a ridiculous idea.

"Every time you smile at someone, it's an action of love,

a gift to that person, a beautiful thing."

~Mother Teresa

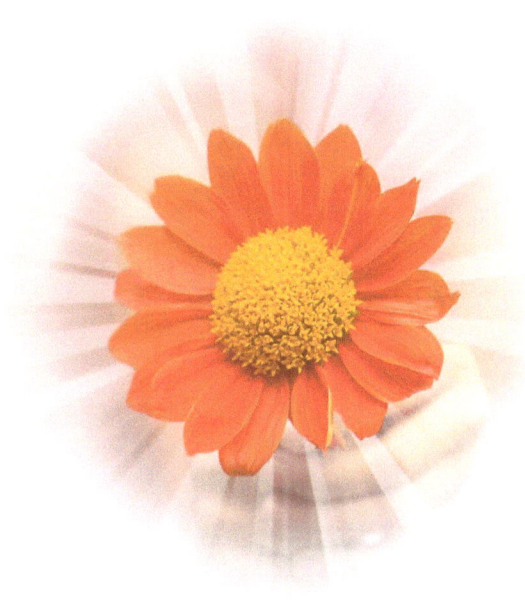

Susan C. Dewey

Chapter Five

FLOWER POWER

I made a unique, eye-opening discovery one day. To share the story, I have to begin by telling you something funny and probably not too interesting about myself, but it's relative to how this incident came to be. I, as a personal rule, do not wear my hair in a ponytail. I do not like how they look on me. Did you ever see one of those apple head dolls they used to make in Girl Scouts? When I put my hair in a ponytail, I feel like a shrunken apple head doll, so I never do it. This particular day I woke up so late for work that I had no choice but to tame this wildly frizzy, curly mop with a dreaded ponytail. It looked so ridiculous, I couldn't bear it. I found a hair clip with a light pink flower on it. I clipped it on the side of my head, and said to myself, "Jeeze, that looks ridiculous, but it looks better than nothing," and walked out the door. I felt silly walking around with my gaudy hair clip and ponytail.

For the past few days, I'd been caring for an elderly COPD patient who was always so mean and literally never had anything nice to say. She hated everyone and everything in the hospital. Every time I came in to give her a nebulizer treatment, she'd snarl, "Oh, it's you again," with her scrunched brow and curled top lip. I'd say, "Good morning, I'm Susan. I am your Respiratory Therapist today and I have a breathing/nebulizer treatment for you this morning." She'd snarl back, "I don't want it, and I'm

33

tired of looking at you, but you're already here, so go on, let's get this over with!" This particular morning, I'll never forget. As usual, I was hesitant about going into her room, preparing for the angry jabs, putting my imaginary rubbery defense up, so the insults would bounce off of me and not get me down. I entered her room, slowly taking a deep breath, but what happened next was miraculous.

I began my introduction, "Good morn-," I was cut off. "I love that flower in your hair!" she exclaimed, with an actual real smile on her face! "Do you have my breathing treatment?" Holy cow! I was speechless. I felt paralyzed for a second or two, thinking to myself, "Did that just happen? Where's my patient and who's this one in her place?" I smiled ear to ear and we began discussing this flower in my hair, laughing about my shrunken apple head story and we ended up sharing a hug after her treatment. I told her I was so glad to see her smiling. How amazing! I returned later in the day for her second treatment and she said she'd been looking forward to it. I literally made her day by pure accident. I thought to myself the next morning, "What if I wear it again? Could I possibly get the same smiling response from her two days in a row?" I sure did! I've worn a flower in my hair every day since.

It's become an ice breaker for some; something to smile about for others. It's prompted patients to tell me the most interesting stories. I've heard many stories from male patients who spend time in Hawaii during their service in the military. They always have a really beautiful story to tell about a beautiful Hawaiian woman and tell me how wearing it on one side or the other signified their marital/dating status. So many smiles have come from this flower of mine. I began discovering how easy it's to make a difference, even if it's as simple as causing my patient to smile. It may be the only time they smile all day. It doesn't always work, but when it does, it feels so good for my spirit as well as my patients'.

I recently had a patient who had injuries involving his eyes, which were swollen shut. I walked into the room and, as I always do, introduced myself and explained why I was there. He'd never had had a nebulizer treatment before, so I explained it to him and, since he couldn't see me, I described step-by-step what I was doing. Funny thing is, that's not what made the difference. He asked me, after I told him he had another treatment at 2:00, "Will you be back? I want you to come back, not someone else." I inquired why because it struck me as odd. He said, "Because you're the first person to come into my room and smile." I paused and re-examined him, I really didn't think he could see me or open his eyes, but maybe he was able to peek through a small opening. I said, "Mr. Jones, are you pulling my leg? You can see me? How do you know I'm smiling?" He said, "I can hear it in your voice." I never really thought about it that way. Of course I knew I was coming back, so I assured him I'd be back and joked with him that I'd spread the word that he prefers pretty, smiling caregivers over old, frumpy, and grouchy ones, and we had a good laugh! When I returned, he was up in his chair with a visitor and he said to his friend, "She's smiling, isn't she? She doesn't believe that I can hear it in her voice." We chatted for a few moments and laughed some more. He asked me if I could be his therapist the next day. I explained that we don't often get the same assignment twice in a row, but that I would come up and say hello to him, which I did.

My patients often ask if they'll have me as their therapist again, but the way we're assigned doesn't make a lot of sense. Getting to know our patients is very important to delivering good care. As we get to know them, we get to know what's normal for them and can spot problems or declining conditions easily and quickly. Unfortunately, it doesn't work that way right now. We're staffed wherever they feel the need to put us. Continuity of care is an important element to consider observing a bit closer. If we've successfully built a trust with our patients, the best option would be to continue that throughout the patient's stay if at all possible.

What happens when we interrupt that trust could be devastating to what we were trying to accomplish. It only takes one little thing by another caregiver to undo the trust we've worked to establish. Since we often only work three 12-hour shifts per week, this does become a challenge, but we need to consider how to better address this challenge. It never fails that we see a patient and the patient or their loved one asks how I think they're doing. Most often, I have to say, "I've never had them as a patient before, so I can't give them a good comparison," but based on what I see has been charted, I do my best to assess whether there's been improvement or not. This brings to mind another hurdle when we have such heavy workloads—we aren't able to look at the patient's chart for recent progress notes, x-rays, or info on procedures the patient has had done. This impacts our ability to give appropriate care in some cases.

"The quality of a person's life is in direct proportion to their commitment to excellence, regardless of their chosen field of endeavor."

~Vince Lombardi

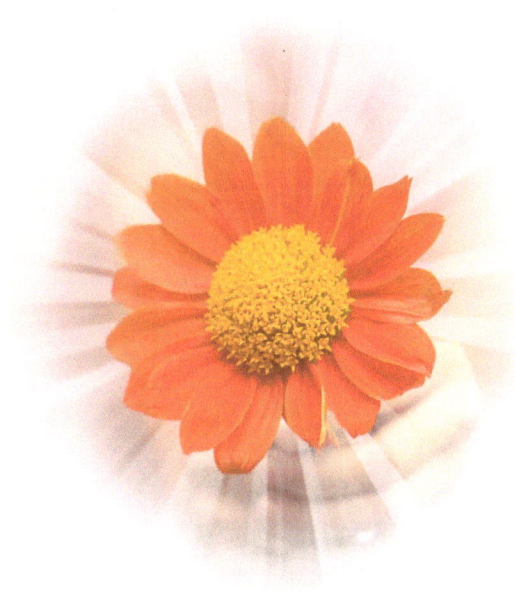

Susan C. Dewey

Chapter Six

WHO CARES?

In the infancy of this project's development, I received a phone call while pondering what to do with these ideas in making a difference in patient care. A former co-worker had called, and I was sharing this project and my ideas with him. He decided to let me know, like he had the day he'd commented on the trach patient in my earlier story, that people don't care, and that what I'm doing won't make a difference. His opinion is that the people we work with don't care enough to change. The disconnect between those of us on the front line and the administrators and CEOs at the top is so great that it won't ever change. His opinion is that the CEOs don't care about people or patients; they only care what they can do to make themselves look good and how much money they make. They say all the right things to make themselves look good, like talking about patient care and patient experience, but in reality, they don't give two hoots about it.

My former co-worker might be right, and that might be the case. But I have a big problem with that attitude because, if someone doesn't try to make a difference, it'll never change. It takes someone to go out and try in order for anything to happen. Will this book change the world? Will it change an entire hospital? Probably not, but can it change one patient's experience? It absolutely can. I'm not putting myself above or saying I'm better than anyone else. I've just learned to treat my patients like human beings, and I care. The mission I'm on is to put the care back in healthcare for all patients. It's been forgotten. Caring has been forgotten in everyday life. If you look at the world around us, people don't care. My coworker was right about that. The work we do, taking care of patients, is so important. We have the ability to make a very bad experience in their life better. Not everyone came into healthcare to help people, I understand that. There are a variety of positions, with better than average pay in some cases, job security, and the number of jobs available make it an attractive career option to many. Not everyone got into healthcare to care about people, but if we're in it now, we need to learn how to connect with our patients and help them feel better so that they may heal. We work our butts off. We're overloaded with patients and work needing to get done. What I've learned is that it doesn't take a lot to make a difference to a patient.

I have ideas and techniques that I find effective, and wish to share them. I know they work because my patients tell me. The fact that they tell me, tells me this. It stands out. It's unusual. Patients are not used to being treated that way. If they were, they wouldn't be mentioning it, and that it made their day better. If it happened all the time, it would be the norm, and they wouldn't feel the need to mention it.

These problems are nationwide. They're not hospital-specific; I'm not singling out any hospital. This is just my collection of observations, ideas, and "ah-ha" moments I've had as I've traveled through my healthcare career. I'm a Registered Respiratory Therapist, I can't speak for nurses or other healthcare departments, but in my role, every day we're given an assignment. Our assignment might be two or three floors and an ICU, sometimes on the opposite side of the hospital. If an ICU is particularly busy, we might get lucky and just have that ICU, but that's rare. Most often we work multiple areas, and we have a heavy workload. The focus is no longer on patient care; it's on numbers and productivity.

What is productivity? Well, everything we do is assigned a value—a point value or minute value. This value system differs from one hospital to another. Every treatment, medication administration, education session, and therapy has a point or minute value assigned. Our assignments are based on a predetermined number of points or minutes we're expected to complete in our shift. If we do not reach our predetermined productivity, it's usually mentioned to us. Often we're questioned to find out why we didn't reach our productivity for the shift. If we want to care about our patient, it could cost us valuable time. If we want to treat our patients as human beings, it takes a little extra time. We're not encouraged to do that. Instead, we're encouraged to get the work done, produce the points or numbers, and reach our productivity.

Let me give you an example of how this works and why I'm saying this. We do patient rounds multiple times a day—giving treatments, performing therapies, doing vent checks, and checking oxygen and trachs. As Respiratory Therapists, we've a two-hour window to get treatments done. A standard nebulizer treatment with one medication takes about 10 minutes, including assessment, if we just do our assessment and the nebulizer. Some treatments consist of up to 5 medications, some of which cannot be mixed; however, you'll still see it done. I was told by another therapist, "I mix them if I need to, whatever makes the treatment faster so I can get them done." Those multiple medication treatments take 25-35 minutes. Now, if I have 30 treatments to give, and often we have 25-30 single-dose nebulizer treatments to do in the morning rounds, it would take 4-5 hours do them appropriately, meaning one-on-one care, one patient at a time. It would take more time if there are a lot of medication combos being given. For those, add at least an hour depending on how many patients have those combos.

So, how do we get the work done, you ask? We do something called stacking treatments. We have to have multiple patients on treatments at a time, which is a big no-no. This is also a great way to overlook important things. How do we find time to understand what's going on with our patients? Often, shift change does not include a detailed report—this has become a problem in many departments. Unless you work in an ICU, you might not get report at all. Even in the ICU, you may not get the information you need to fully see the clinical picture of your patients and their conditions. And if we run around doing 4-5 hours of work in 2-3 hours, when do you think we have time to read the chart notes or progress notes? Exactly! We don't.

To deliver quality one-on-one care, there's no possible way to deliver more than 12-18 single-dose treatments in a 2-3 hour window. Is 10 minutes each a reasonable amount of time to consider per treatment? Well, we enter, introduce ourselves, check the patient identity, scan or check the meds to be given, listen to lung sounds, check heart rate and respiratory rate, and then begin the nebulizer, which runs for a minimum of 8 minutes for one dose of one med. Some hospitals have gone to a high-flow nebulizer, which literature says can deliver a full single dose or 3ml in 3 minutes. If we use that as our nebulizer in the previous example, I would say it's reasonable to consider we could complete approximately 20 treatments in two hours. That's still only assuming we're giving our patient minimum attention. Some of the specialty medications cannot be nebulized 3 minutes, so we have to consider that as well. We go about our business with the usual approach, and if our patients don't need any attention, or have any other needs or questions, then we're not too far off. If we want to care about our patients, connect on the human level, and establish trust it will add a minimum of at least a few minutes to each treatment. Some patients have never had nebulizer treatments before and need information, education, and instruction. They may need questions answered as well, so add time for that.

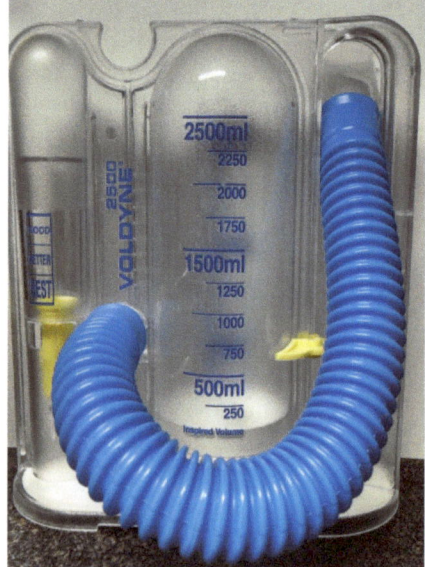

Some patients are given therapies to perform and have not been properly instructed. I recently had a patient with very high oxygen needs; so high in fact, it was difficult for her to imagine how she would go home with that type of oxygen need. I asked if she had ever used an Incentive Spirometer (pictured), a device that, when used correctly, simulates the deep breaths we take when we're up and walking, doing our regular daily routines.

When patients are ill and off their feet, this therapy can help them avoid pneumonia and atelectasis, reversing the effects of both. This therapy opens up the lungs, allowing improved oxygenation, and stimulates removal of secretions by stimulating coughing. This patient proudly told me that she had one at home and could reach the maximum 2500ml on it. I knew from looking at her and her small frame, and the fact that she already has home oxygen, that she probably wasn't doing it correctly. I gave her an IS and asked her to show me how she was using it at home. Sure enough, no one ever taught her how to use it. She said, "No, they just brought it in and set it down on my table and told me to use it." After instructing her on proper technique, I gave her a few hours to practice. I returned to her room on my next round. Her oxygen need was cut in half just by using the device properly with correct technique. My time with her on the first visit took 30 minutes. Was it worth it? What's your opinion? In my opinion, these are the types of interactions that build the connections and trust with our patients, and are simply the right thing to do. This patient's outcome and risk of re-admission are greatly affected by the interaction I had with her, and she's now armed with the knowledge of how to help her respiratory status and reduce oxygen requirements. This is patient care!

Nurses have similar problems with patient ratios and the number of medications they have to deliver to each patient. This causes a competition for time with the patient, but not quality time. Who gets to go first? The nurse, x-ray, lab, or the therapist? Does it support a positive experience for our patients, or our staff? As a result, the mindset has changed. People don't care; we *can't* care. If you take the time to care about a patient, you're not going to have the productivity at an acceptable level, and one of your superiors will question you about it. When we work in healthcare and we want to take care of patients and treat them like people, like human beings, it's very difficult to watch our coworkers not care, and work side-by-side with people who don't care. Deep down, I believe they wish they could, and once did. We've adapted, we've turned it off. We've become indifferent and are getting their work done. We don't take the time to do what's right for our patient. I've taken the time to do what's right for my patient and in multiple different hospitals, multiple different departments and managers, and I've been told all three times, "Stop wasting your time. That's not your job; you need to get your work done." I beg to differ. If I have the skills and the ability to take care of the needs of a patient, I should be allowed to do it. It's my job. It's everyone's job. That's patient care. That extra time we take could mean the difference in the patient's outcome.

"The task of the leader is to get his people from where they are to where they have not been."

~Henry A. Kissinger

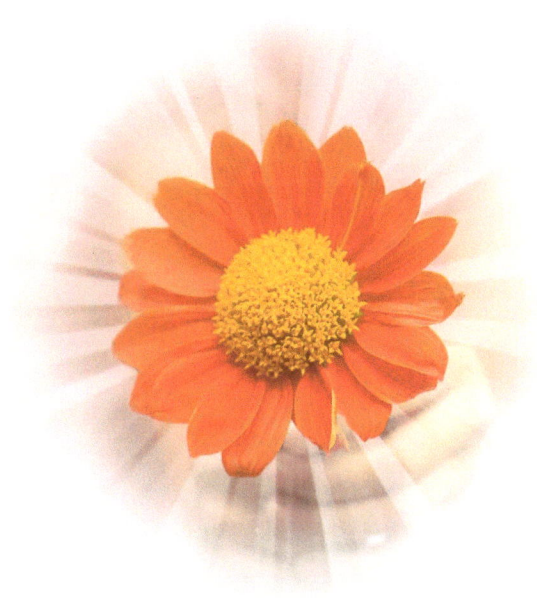

Susan C. Dewey

Chapter Seven

ANALYZING PATIENT CARE

We're working in a system and with an approach that's been used for over 50 years. Fifty years ago, it probably worked very well. You might be asking yourself, what's changed? We've got more patients than we've ever had before. But we've got a population that has more sickness and chronic disease than we've ever seen before. We perform more medical and surgical miracles than we ever have before. The advances in medicine and surgical procedures bring more patients to our hospitals, and we perform miracles in our hospitals and facilities every day. We save lives, but we're not allowed to care. This creates quite a challenge to return to work every day and feel even close to fulfilled if we can't take care of people like they're human beings and care about them.

We hear so much these days about patient experience and patient satisfaction. Hospitals are paid by Medicare based on patient satisfaction scores. We have Patient Experience Directors and Patient Experience Vice Presidents. Do you know what they do? They crunch numbers. They're data analysts. I don't think they get it. I believe the solution could be found by talking to our patients. Rounding on our patients, asking them, "What are we doing right?" "What needs to be better?" "How do you feel your care could be better?" "What's working, what's not?" When you get your patient input, you then work backward to step two. Go to your staff.

This point is when and where you can ask, why is this happening? What's causing these failures? Is the administration in your facility even aware of the current ratios you and your staff are managing? What processes or ideas lead to this success? Maybe there's a central supply issue causing backordered items in dire need by your staff to perform the needed care. Could there be a medication shortage causing dear Aunt Sally's complaint about not getting the medications she needs or knows she's supposed to have? Is it an equipment problem? Are we short on supplies? It could be anything, but how do we know if we're trying to solve this problem sitting in an office crunching numbers instead of asking the patients and our staff members? That's where the solutions lie to patient satisfaction. When we stop looking at numbers and go back to looking at patients and caring, our patient satisfaction scores will improve by default.

"If everyone is moving forward together,

then success takes care of itself."

~Henry Ford

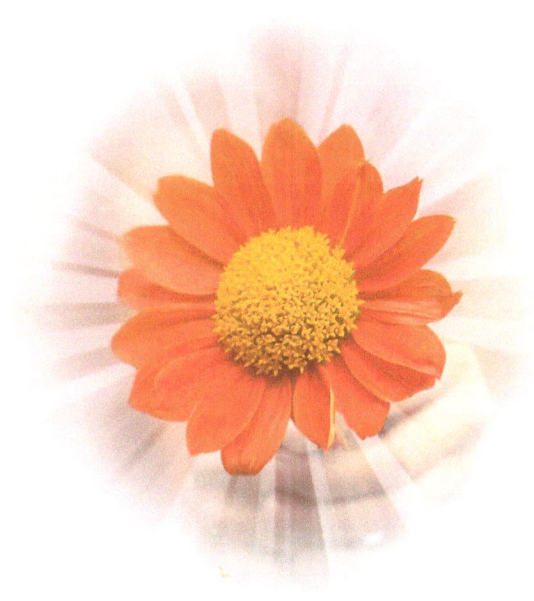

Chapter Eight

CREDENTIALS ARE USELESS IF WE DON'T CARE

When I started this adventure of making a difference in patient care, I started doing research. I read a lot of books, listened to speakers, and attended conferences all on patient care and how to improve it. What made such a difference was hearing other people express in detail the same ideas and thoughts that I have. CEOs and designated staff conducting patient rounds, finding solutions to the indifference that plagues our staff, including the patients and staff in concepts for solutions, and getting back to doing fulfilling work. They have successfully made the changes I have tried to suggest over and over.

The differences between myself and the people I read about and listen to, are the degrees we hold, the letters after our names. That's not how they were successful in their patient care mission. They were successful because of what we have in common. We care about people. We care about our patients, their care and their experiences in our care. That's the *only* way to make a difference— to care. They wanted what I want: to do work that's fulfilling, to do something worthwhile. During the process of improving their patients' experience, they discovered that, without knowing it, they were also improving their patient satisfaction scores. There is your proof: If we go back to caring about our patients, caring about people, the numbers follow by default. Not only that, but it also improves the morale of their staff. By going back to the basics of taking care of people, you don't have to crunch numbers anymore. The numbers take care of themselves. It doesn't require special abbreviations after your name to make a difference. ALL IT TAKES IS SOMEONE WHO CARES!

What is the first step in improving how we care for our patients? Connecting with them is the first step. As human beings we can sense when someone is being genuine, and as human beings so can our patients. Connecting is not speaking predetermined, scripted messages. It is speaking as if we are speaking to another human being, not an object. Why do many speeches not strike us as they are meant to? They lack the component that connects the speaker to the audience — sincerity. The first step is smiling and making eye contact when we approach our patients. A genuine smile can create a connection between any two people. We are pretty good at the script, "Good morning Mr.____, my name is _____ I am a_____ I am here to give you or administer your_____." At that point, we go about our business as just that, business. When in reality, continuing to connect is what we should be doing. By continuing we are able to lay the ground work for establishing the patient's trust.

A number of hospitals use different programs to achieve trust from their patients, but the simple fact is, they don't work. It's up to each staff member to establish a personal connection and trust from their patients. These programs simply give your staff another thing to focus on besides the patient. I once worked at a hospital that used trust cards and trust huddles as part of their patient experience program. What does this do? It takes them away from their work to attend a discussion in which they already have no interest. They're not interested because it comes from administrators who are disconnected from the frontline, bedside staff. They have now successfully taken more valuable time out of their employees' day, allowing even less time to get the work done.

In any situation we encounter, how do we establish trust? For starters, if you say you're going to do something, do it. And do it intentionally. The opportunity to build trust with our patients is priceless. When we fail to follow through, the person counting on us learns they absolutely can't count on us. Trust is lost. If a patient asks you for a blanket, can you get it? Most of us won't because we're focused on getting to the next patient. If you tell the patient you can't, or it's not your job, they get frustrated, which causes a negative patient experience. You've let them down. If you really can't, it's better to say something to the effect of, "I'm new here, and don't know exactly where the blankets are, but I can find someone to get one for you." If you are unable to do something that's asked of you, there's someone who probably can. Find them! Make sure it gets handled! The patient is at everyone's mercy. They are not usually allowed to get up and wander around to find a blanket or drink of water. They depend and count on us to meet their needs, so if you say you're going to do something, do it.

Co-workers who follow me on night shift get very upset that I put my phone number on the patient's white board. I put it there when I'm connecting with them and building trust. After I begin their nebulizer treatment, I tell them that if they need anything, to give me a call. I point out that my number is on their board and tell them that it's there for them to use. I let them know that while I may not be able to be there right away, but if I can't get there, I'll make sure someone else is. I have to say this because if you work in healthcare, you know a code blue can ruin every promise you made to patients that day, so I always let them know that sometimes things come up, but if I can't make it, I will send someone. Co-workers don't like this because they don't want their phone ringing and patients calling. The reality is, when you use this technique, the patients rarely call. When they do, it's for something important like they are short of breath. To be honest, I haven't had a patient call me for anything non-emergent yet. Sometimes, I have visiting loved ones call me, and when I arrive, I just increased their level of trust. Just offering that to your patients makes them feel more at ease.

David Feinberg, CEO of UCLA Health System, has taken this a step further and rebuilt trust in the physicians and surgeons as well as administrative staff. Patients are rounded on daily by himself, key administrators, and the physicians and surgeons involved in their case. Patients receive their business card with a

24-hour, 7-days a week number to reach them. Every single one of them. One would immediately think that patients would abuse this opportunity, but they don't.

However, how helpful is it when a patient doesn't understand something and a loved one needs to speak with a doctor to understand the patient's condition or outlook? It's a useful tool in building trust with our patients and increasing patient satisfaction because they have had a highly positive patient experience. This concept also makes our administrators and doctors accountable for what happens in our hospitals, and arms them with the information they need to make effective changes. When David Feinberg returned his hospital's focus to the patient and finding solutions, aided by the front line staff, a number of things happened. The hospitals patient satisfaction scores began rising quickly from the 30th percentile to the 90th. Not only did patient satisfaction scores improve, so did the morale of his staff. He explained in one of his presentations that they now have employees who feel like they are doing work that matters, that's fulfilling. As a result, one job opening for an RN is known to bring 3,000-4,000 applicants. They also chose to use a screening tool called Talent Plus, developed as a tool to find and maximize human potential. It helps find the applicants who are driven to make a difference and deliver better patient care.

I've been asked, "Isn't it just good customer service?" Well, I can say that if you treated your customers the way we should be treating our patients you would have a booming business. We're not just serving customers; we're making human connections and delivering human experiences, not customer service. Can it be applied to business? Yes. In every business, a genuine human connection built on trust and caring will result in a thriving business, no matter the type.

"If your actions inspire others to dream more, learn more, do more and become more, you are a leader."

~John Quincy Adams

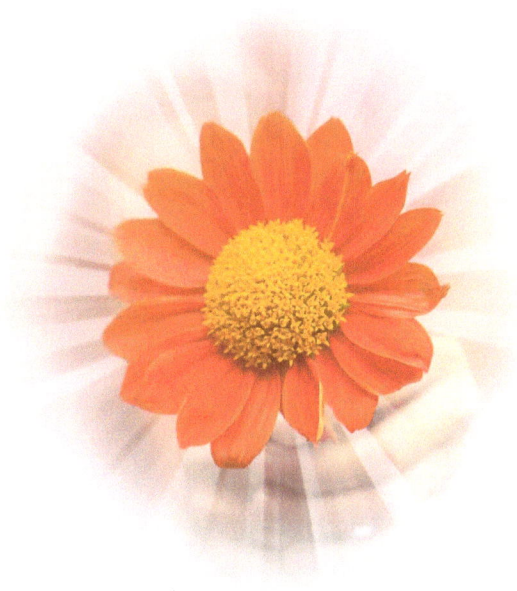

Susan C. Dewey

Chapter Nine

THE RIPPLE EFFECT

I have seen so many things that are wrong in my hospital travels that I used to wonder, "What if 'they' could see and really know what goes on at the bedside, the frontline?"—'they' being the CEOs and administrators who dream up these magnificent but useless programs for our staff to improve patient experience. If they talked to our patients, if even I could round on patients, which was my original idea, then maybe I could make a difference and have a voice that could be heard.

I've been turned down numerous times. What I knew was that they just never "got it." They can't see what we see. We see the successes and the failures that affect human lives. They see numbers. I felt the answer to bridging the gap was initiating patient rounding by someone, anyone, who cared. David Feinberg had the same idea I had, and put it into practice. That was when I said to myself, "I'm onto something here." This guy saw what I see, he was in a position to make it happen, and the results were outstanding. What made him successful? Was it his CEO status, the letters MD after his name? No. What made him successful was that he cared about people, and doing the right thing for his patients. He was a man who found fulfillment in helping others. He was motivated to do meaningful work. Many of us are driven by the same passion, but are shut down and ignored because we lack certain letters before or after our names. I declare though, that it's possible. It's often the actions of one person that begins the ripple of change.

We do have many success stories in our hospitals. We have many happy patient stories. We have fantastic nurses and staff who work very hard and do a good job. It's difficult, however, in our current approach to be successful. As I said earlier, we have angels disguised as nurses touching lives every day. I think we could find more of those angels if we took the right steps to change the way we work and care for our patients. If we could unite our team of caregivers, including our physicians and surgeons, and put our patients first, we could see results that no one ever could have imagined.

Another way to build trust is in our team. Doctors listening to clinical staff about medications and therapies—reducing the number of unnecessary medications or therapies would save our staff valuable time. Training our doctors properly on electronic ordering, just as we do the rest of our staff, would save time that I spent calling and paging physicians to get orders corrected. This is not the fault of the physicians, but rather our system that doesn't recognize how big the problem is. Many hospitals are teaching hospitals, and our residents are not well-versed in our ordering systems. It is not possible to modify or change an order without the doctor's consent, so it's very important to build this vital part of our team as well. Too many of our physicians are permitted to order staff around and behave as if they are above the rest. I've been shouted at over the phone because a doctor was scrubbed in for surgery and had to return my page. I had to page him because he ordered a medication for a patient, but ordered it incorrectly. Until I'd had it corrected, I couldn't give this patient anything, but I was being reprimanded for causing this doctor's inconvenience.

We are often discouraged from making suggestions to them. They believe they know best. I was a new employee at one hospital and was flying solo during my first night shift after orientation. Surprisingly, I was given the charge therapist phone, and received a call for a STAT EKG in the OR (operating room). My first hurdle: I didn't know where OR was located. I was able to find it with a little help, arrived in the pre-op area looking for my patient. Come to find out, they were already on the operating table and this EKG was supposed to be done hours ago, on the day shift, so no one was happy to see me. I put my leads on the patient and found a slight issue in the software configuration. It was not set up for OR and I couldn't pull the patient up in the EKG system.

The anesthesiologist began slamming me, "What's taking so long? Don't you know how to do your effing job?" I was doing all I could to pull the patient up as fast as I could. He yelled, "What's the effing problem? Hurry up! We're in the OR, you know! I could do it faster than you! Are you an effing idiot?" That was the moment I turned around and said, "Well sir, this is my first day here, I also work at two other hospitals where they're happy to have me. I can go home right now. So, if you can do this faster than me, you go right ahead! Otherwise, please stop shouting at me!" I was trembling because I'd never spoken to a doctor that way. I was also angry that he thought he could abuse me that way. He told me just to pick any patient name and get on with the EKG, and the powers that be could fix it in the morning and to tell them doctor "so and so" told me to do it. I did. And I was more than inclined to include all the details of what led up to the patient name mix up. However, nothing was ever done about it. They weren't going to speak to the doctor because he is "The Doctor". Come to find out, it's also policy in that hospital that EKGs in the OR are only done by OR nurses, not by the Respiratory Department. OMG! I wanted to scream! If we're going to work as a team, this type of superiority complex has to be addressed. We're here to collaborate with each other for the sake of our patient and providing their best outcome. It's a vital part of patient care and improving patients' experience.

Many employees feel like pawns under the control of administrators and physicians. We see what is best for the patient and what is not working or causing them to decline. In reality we're the front line staff who holds the key to the best solutions. Just as in a battle, no one knows the conditions on the battlefield better than those fighting on it. The men on the frontlines report opportunities to advance, casualties and successes to the generals who report on up the chain. The front line is not ignored or treated as insignificant. Our health systems work backwards in this respect. The CEOs and administration send orders down the chain to the front line, who end up working with processes and policies that cause more harm than good. When we use processes that don't work, we lose time we could spend with our patients. Those processes are often left in place not addressing the fact that they aren't working. Our administrators and CEOs, I believe, have the best intentions when coming up with new processes and policies, but they've never worked at the patients' bedside, or haven't done so in so long, they truly are disconnected from what is happening and what challenges we face.

In a recent conversation with a nurse manager, she voiced frustration concerning how we work. She said, "I took this position, this promotion to be a leader. I'm so busy doing paper work and chasing software problems I don't get to function as a leader. I wanted to be able to make my nurses' work fulfilling again, so they feel like they're doing something that matters." I found this very applicable to the problems my department faces. Many of us have a desire to lead and make a difference, but we're dismissed as insignificant because of our degrees and those abbreviations before or after our names. If you are not aware of and utilizing the people on your staff who are motivated to be leaders and determined to go above and beyond for our patients, you're not an effective leader. Those staff members have ideas and suggestions that come from firsthand experience. When administrators and physicians ignore them, they feel underappreciated and devalued.

We must not continue practicing indifference within our leadership. The most valuable ideas for solutions have historically come from small groups of people with similar goals. I've seen a hospital utilize its staff in a collaborative way to significantly reduce VAP (ventilator acquired pneumonia) and UTIs (urinary tract infections) to levels so low they were nationally recognized, and other facilities have now instituted the same policies and protocols. It was not a CEO or administrator who decided what to do. It was the members of staff who work on our frontlines, the staff members whose ideas were taken into consideration and tested. This approach is a win-win for staff, administration, and the patients.

Not all of the staff is motivated to be leaders, or go the extra mile for their patients. Some don't care about feeling fulfilled by their work and maybe they never will care. There may be staff members who need to be let go because they are not suited for patient care. Quint Studer, Founder of the Studer Group and author of *Hardwiring Excellence*, entered into healthcare from corporate America and turned a nearly failing hospital into a successful one by refocusing on the patients. In his book, "Hardwiring Excellence" he outlines the difficulties he faced: staff are often reluctant to change or to welcome change to their work. When considering such radical changes, it's realistic to consider the likelihood that there will be resistance, but he proved it's possible to resurrect a hospital and its falling morale. He uses phrases that I find very poignant, such as evidence-based leadership.

If you work in healthcare, you know we already used evidence-based practice, sometimes called evidence-based medicine. Mr. Studer takes it a step further to introduce evidence-based leadership. It's his way of aligning the care/medicine with the leadership, according to Mr. Studer it is a "correlation of best practices and consistency of leadership practices." He was the first executive to use the exact same terms I use when thinking about the issues and solutions. I read his book twice because I couldn't believe someone thought the same way I did, to the extent of using the same phrases. Quint Studer and David Feinberg have already proven that the things I discuss are possible and will work when an organization is dedicated to improvement. Could it mean letting employees go that are not on board or are resistant to change and refuse to take part? Yes. Will these employees be replaced by better-suited candidates who are eager to make a difference? Yes.

Susan C. Dewey

"To pay attention, this is our endless and proper work."
~Mary Oliver

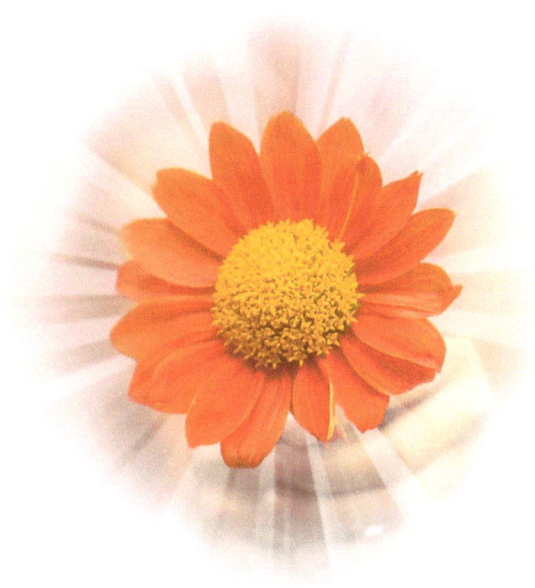

Susan C. Dewey

Chapter Ten

YOU HAVE TO BE PAYING ATTENTION TO PAY ATTENTION

When I look around at many workplaces, I see things right away that could be quick, simple fixes that make a huge impact on patient care and patient experience. They directly influence the overall public view of some hospitals and facilities. The first, I cannot stress enough how important it is: Your staff needs to disconnect from mobile devices while in work areas. I was visiting a facility for some meetings and immediately took notice of all the people walking down the halls smiling, and telling me good morning, asking if I needed assistance finding my way. Every one of them either smiled or greeted me. No matter which they did, they made eye contact with me in a welcoming manner. The contrast between this experience and so many others I've had at other facilities emphasized the fact that we should never see staff walking down hallways or standing at desks looking at their mobile device.

Let's begin with the doctors. The argument can be made that, since we've moved to an electronic ordering system and medical record, doctors should be allowed to use their mobile devices in any place because they're often on them putting orders in or responding to patient-related electronic messages. What did doctors do before mobile devices? They had a paging system which required them to find a telephone to return the page. If it required details about patients they often ducked into an office for privacy. This could still be done. Remove mobile devices from patient and visitor areas. Physicians can use an office to address issues on their mobile devices, just as they did before. Why is this important? Because the mentality goes that if the physicians can have their mobile device out, so can I. To reel this idea in, everyone should be on the same playing field. Same expectations. Does it matter? How does it affect our patient care? First of all, it's incredibly rude and inconsiderate. If you are looking down at your phone, you are not looking where you are going. You are not able to notice patients or visitors who need assistance. It causes us to be preoccupied, and we begin to miss important things. It adds to the problem of indifference.

When we're in more of a hurry to reply to a message or see what's happening on social media, mistakes are made and important issues are overlooked. There's a reason that not long ago, mobile devices were not allowed in patient areas. Now they are rampant. They simply provide another distraction from patient care. Sometimes it's crucial to keep work and personal lives separate. We need to be focused on our patients, not our personal problems. Being tethered to our personal life on a mobile device does not lend itself to that. We've to be able to spot a patient in decline and make split second decisions without being preoccupied. It affects our attitudes and perspective and affects our patient's perspective. It's sometimes difficult to not bring our personal lives and problems to work with us, but by having continuous access to it through mobile devices makes it more difficult to move past. How can your employees and physicians see a patient or visitor in need if they can't even see the one in their way? The result is a missed chance to offer direction or assistance that could create a connection and an experience. Some days, even a simple smiling hello can make a difference. That doesn't happen when we're looking down. The only reason to be looking down is to pick someone or something up.

"Science may have found a cure for most evils;

but it has found no remedy for the worst of them all –

the apathy of human beings."

~Helen Keller

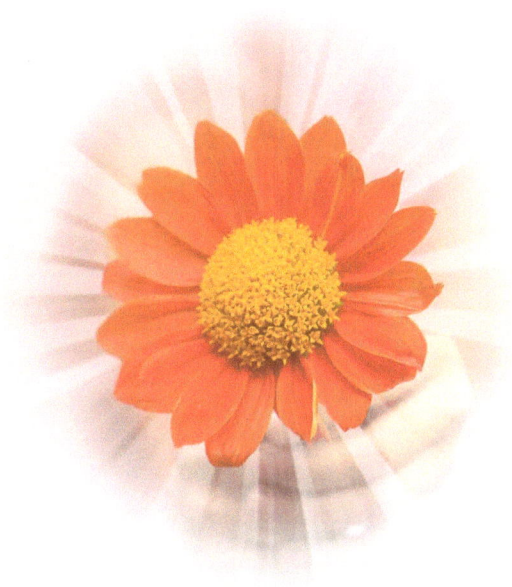

Susan C. Dewey

Chapter 11

IS ANYBODY IN THERE?

Our healthcare system has done a pretty good job in the realm of privacy. HIPAA has helped with that and the long standing efforts to get our staff to comply. When we think about privacy we forget about our patients' personal privacy sometimes. Is there any reason to leave a door or curtain open when bathing a patient? Some of our patients would be horrified if they knew they were lying naked and exposed for all to see. It's human nature to stare and see what's going on, so why not consider your patient's dignity and maintain privacy in these instances as well?

How often have you been a patient and had 6-8 hospital staff join you in the elevator? How do you or would you feel about that? Why isn't it a measure of respect and privacy that patients be transported in an elevator designated solely for them? If I come out of a procedure or test, I would like that common courtesy given to me. I've worked in a number of hospitals where that's a monitored policy. I believe that all hospitals would benefit from adopting the same policy. It benefits your patient and is good practice. It may not seem important, but patients don't often appreciate the small talk of staff, or just the looks from staff while being transported. They feel like they're on display. Another reason this is a good idea is that, if a patient looks unconscious or sedated, we don't whether they can hear us or not. If this is the case, often comments are made that shouldn't be.

I have another short story to demonstrate the importance of this. I was working in an ICU and needed to secure a patient's breathing tube with another device. Another therapist came to lend an extra set of hands. I called the patient by name and told them what we were doing. I immediately noticed grimacing on her face and a tear running down her cheek when we began removing the tape from the patient's cheeks. My co-worker was trying to be comforting and began telling the patient we were trying to be gentle and it that would be over shortly, when at that point my fellow RT blurted out, "Is this a man or a woman?" I couldn't believe it! I replied, "I can't believe you said that! Look at the mani/pedi!" I know they were trying to help and be comforting, but we automatically assume the patient can't hear us. Why? It seemed clear to me that this patient was semi-awake due to her facial expressions and the tear I saw escape her eye. Sometimes we need to stop and think before we speak. If I heard that about myself, I'd want to jump out of my skin! This is why I say that patients are human beings. They feel the same as you and I do. I knew she could hear us, and there was no way to undo what my co-worker had done. I understand that we get busy and have adapted to getting the work done. Why can't we do something to fix this? Let me ask you, would you ask someone at Starbucks or the shopping mall if they were a man or a woman? NO! Most of us would not. It's rude and insensitive. Why would we do it in a hospital to a patient who is already suffering?

When I was still completing my clinical education, I was taking care of an intubated patient, talking to him while I was doing what I needed to do. A family member was there and she asked me if I thought he could hear me. I wasn't sure what to say. I didn't know if he could hear me, which is what I told her. She asked why I was talking to him if I didn't think he could hear me. I said I didn't know. Because honestly, we don't know. I told her I was doing it just in case he could. I'd rather try to put him at ease if I could and let him know what's going on instead of just ignoring the fact that it's possible he could hear me. She said no one had done that before. I thought surely someone had, maybe just not while she was there. I will never forget that woman or the profound impact that conversation had on how I talk to patients, especially my sedated or unconscious patients. Even if I'm just moving the vent tubing to put a nebulizer in line, I always tell them what I'm doing. I figure if they can hear me, it has to be absolutely terrifying to be in their position, unable to communicate or see what's going on around them. So just in case, if it were me, I'd like someone to talk to me so I know what's happening.

Susan C. Dewey

"A little thought and a little kindness are often worth more than a great deal of money."

~John Ruskin

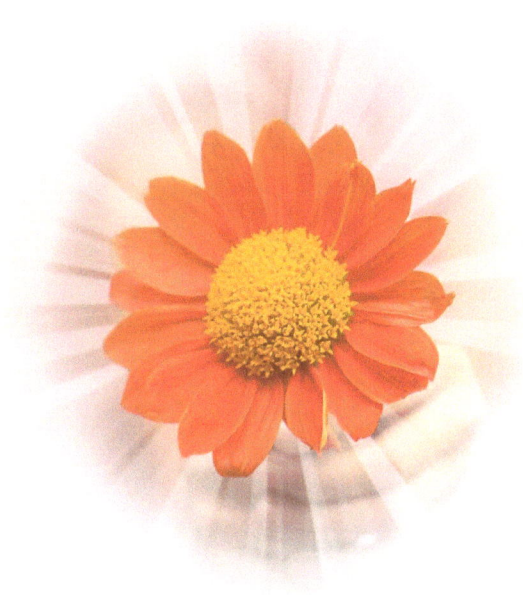

Susan C. Dewey

Chapter 12

THE COST OF CARING

Many hospitals have great policies and protocols in place that protect patients and work to prevent hospital acquired infections. They used evidence based practice to determine what would work and what did work. I can't impress upon hospitals that haven't done this how incredibly important it's to do so. From policies on changing equipment, how to prevent VAP (ventilator associated pneumonia), urinary tract infections from catheter use, and C. diff, staph infections, to reducing the number of patients falling, each one is important and makes a difference when executed appropriately. Policies and protocols dictate how each staff member is expected to perform a task, and leaves no room for indifference.

If we take equipment changes, for example, let me point out that some hospitals don't have policies on when we replace nebulizers, vent circuits, or trach equipment. It's vital that equipment be cleaned, or changed on a regular basis to reduce infection rates. Some patients use the same equipment through their entire stay without it being changed or cleaned. Does it increase costs to change out equipment? Of course it does. We must ask, what are the benefits? Working without policies for equipment leaves us open to cross-contamination and leads to poor patient outcomes. It was estimated in an article from the

Journal of the American Medical Association, that nosocomial infections (aka hospital-acquired infections) cost facilities approximately $9 billion each year. The most common being surgical site infections, ventilator-associated pneumonia, central line infections, and catheter-associated urinary tract infections. This is why policies and protocols related to equipment are vital.

These are ventilators leaving the equipment room and are considered clean and put in use on a patient. It's far from clean and appropriate for use. One could argue that this piece never touches the patient, but the ventilator tubing sits in these holders, and when the patient is turned or repositioned so is the tubing, meaning a nurse, RT or tech is taking the tubing out of the holder, adjusting its position, and returning it to the holder in the new position.

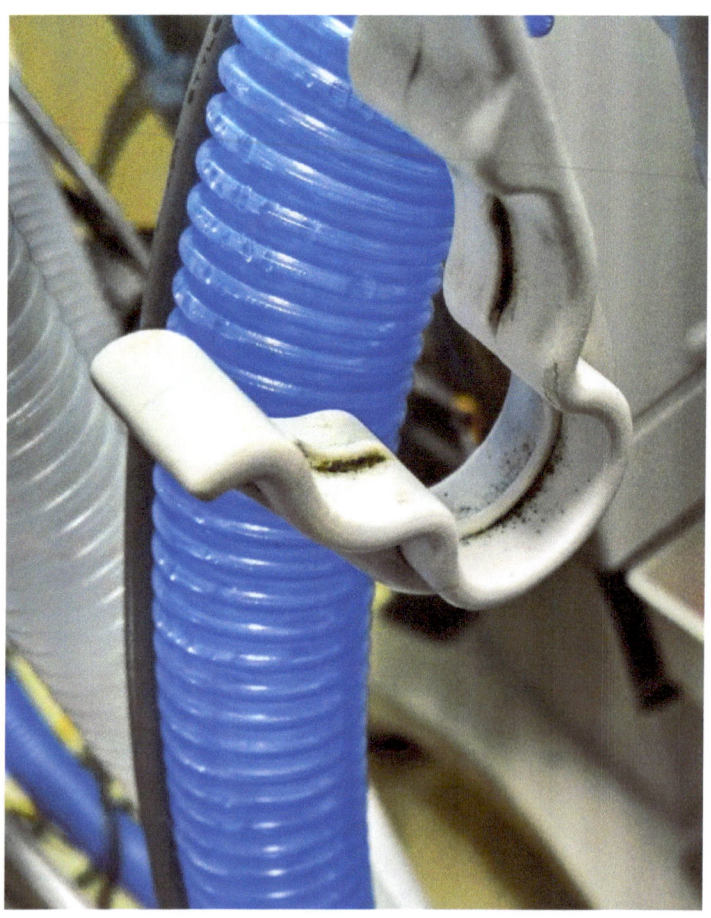

The tubing is contaminated and so are the gloves of the person who made the adjustment. Now whatever they touch is contaminated. No one noticed? Most likely someone noticed, but no one took the time to do anything about it. Most, but not all, facilities have policies for equipment cleaning and changes. There

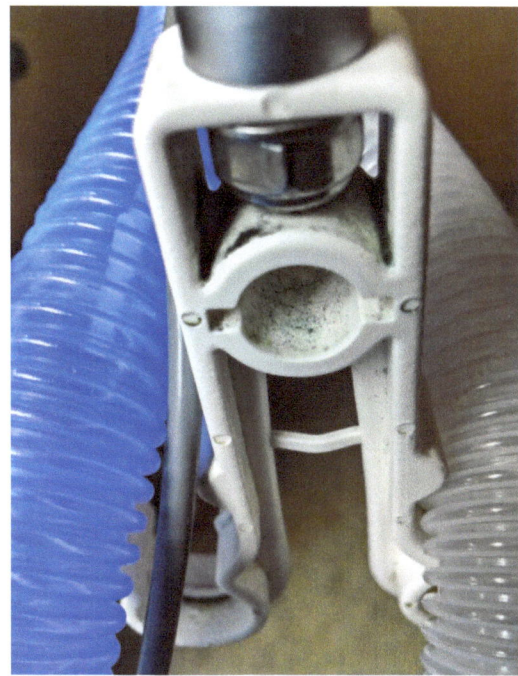

is a point when patient safety outweighs the cost of changing equipment. If your hospital is trying to save money by not using disposable equipment when it can, it could be suffering increased costs from hospital acquired infections. The cost of nosocomial infections is well beyond the cost of creating new policies and procedures and having the ability to be throwing away soiled parts. If we're not able to get over the cost of doing the right thing, our patients will continue to suffer and our patient satisfaction scores will continue to remain where they are instead of improving and climbing.

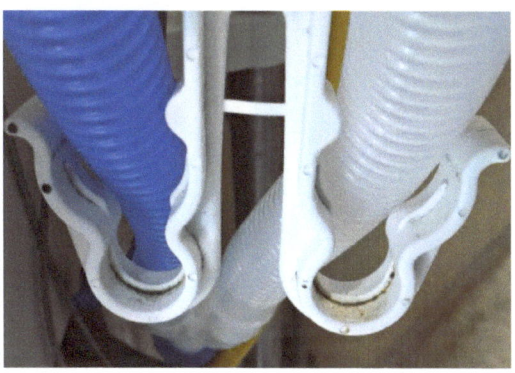

The following pictures depict moldy heated ventilator circuits in use on a patient.

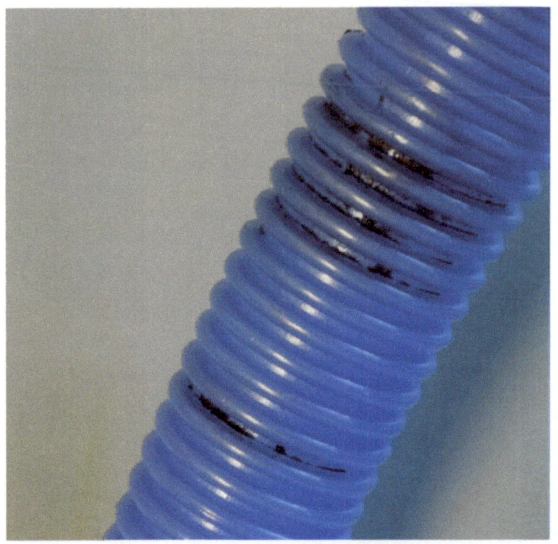

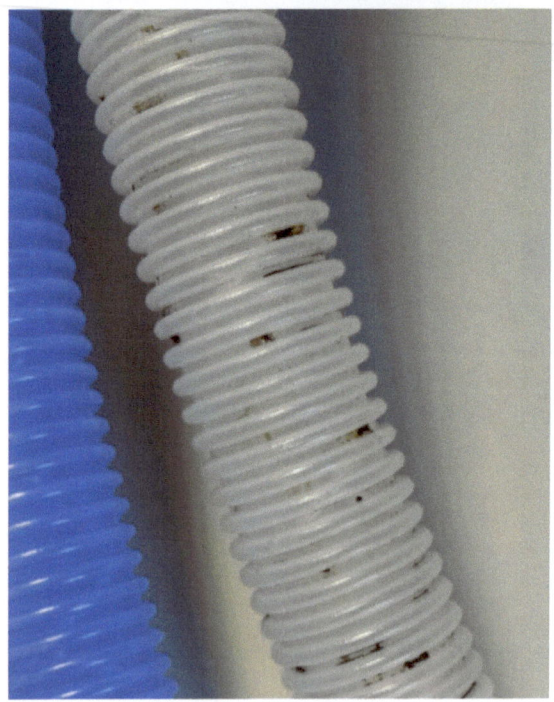

"The empty vessel makes the loudest sound."

~William Shakespeare

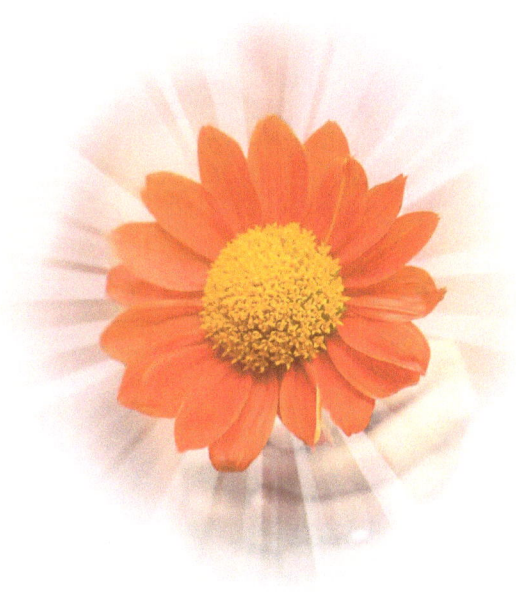

Susan C. Dewey

Chapter 13

SPIRITUAL JOURNEYS

I never realized the depth of how I could care about the work I do until I began working for a large trauma center. I started out just working the assignments I was given and feeling thankful I had a job. As in most respiratory departments, there are those who always complain about their assignments, and those who just deal with the cards they were dealt. Working in a large medical center, we all had heavy workloads and getting that one awful assignment could just start you off on the wrong foot. I began taking notice of which assignment other therapists despised the most—it was the trauma step-down floor, a floor patients are transferred to after leaving the trauma ICU. With heavy patient loads, the trauma floor is a challenge due to the number of trach patients that are part of our assignment. It made a demanding shift just a little hairier.

I had worked the trauma floor numerous times myself. I began to find a kind of inspiration among the traumatic stories I cared for there. When we worked trauma we were usually also given the palliative care floor. Palliative care is end of life care, comfort care. What I never expected was the way I would be transformed. I began electing to take the trauma floor, and made it "my floor" so to speak. It's a place where an awakening happens. A new awareness and new perspective become clear. It isn't just a life that is lost in these tragedies. What is lost is the human spirit — the character, energy and spunk- the life force that make us human beings. When patients suffer brain injuries, whether from an MVA, an overdose, or a fall, the person you once saw in someone's eyes is gone. When families hang up pictures of your patient in their room, I always felt that they did it to try and spark memories. To see a glimpse in their eyes of who they once were. While I worked the night shift, I was often alone with my patients in their room among all those pictures. It was a feeling I never felt before; a grief, a loss, a sadness that can't be described.

I could begin to understand how the families felt, even though I never knew their loved one until they became my patient. Seeing pictures of the human spirit, housed in these bodies which are our vessels, and then seeing the vessel abandoned, empty, not even a glimmer in their eyes, made my heart sink, and tears form in my eyes. The loss of that person that was so full of life was confusing and heartbreaking. In that experience on the trauma floor, I learned how precious our loved ones are. I became much more cautious in my actions, and more protective of my loved ones. Watching a mother or father, sometimes children, talk to my patient, begging them to come back, to wake up, to return to the vessel they left behind, was personal and poignant. Some shifts were filled with overwhelming emotion, but being there and being part of the experience with the families made it impossible to be indifferent. There was no way to avoid being engulfed in the emotion and not feel compelled to comfort them.

Working in trauma was also the experience that taught me about miracles. Some of our patients have suffered such severe trauma, including severe brain injuries that we, along with our patients' loved ones, feel as if there is no hope for recovery. Sometimes the doctors can't even believe it! I recently used this experience to give hope to one family I encountered. They talked as if their loved one could never recover. She was so close to death, and battling numerous severe infections that seemed to impede every step in the right direction. I took about 30 minutes every time I rounded on this patient to talk with the family and keep their hope alive. I told them of my experiences working in trauma units. I told them they could never give up hope, because even I've been surprised at the recoveries I've seen in my trauma experience. I've seen patients who have survived as empty vessels like the ones I described earlier. I've seen patients overcome severe infections. I've seen miraculous recoveries from patients in the most hopeless and traumatic situations. If the family gives up hope, why wouldn't their loved one give up as well? Some time went by and I hadn't seen this family in a few months, but I knew their loved one was still a patient in our care. I recently noticed the patient had been moved to another area of the hospital that I regularly cover and was assigned to this day. I entered a room that was filled with energy and laughter. My patient was talking and laughing, and was about to have their trach removed permanently. The mother winked at me and said, "She is a miracle!". I smiled and winked back. These are the rewards we depend on to keep coming back every day. Experiences such as these fill our hearts with hope and give meaning to what we do.

The same was true on the palliative care unit. When families have to make a decision for their loved ones to end their suffering it can be extremely emotional. The range of feelings goes from sadness, to doubt, to grief. Sometimes something happens that restores hope in the family that their loved one can come back, so they struggle with doing the right thing. What is the right thing? That is the struggle. They question themselves and examine their conscience and try to do what their dying loved one would want them to do, most of the time without a living will or advanced directive, which makes it a tormenting experience on top of all the other emotions. When it came down to it, families looked to us for guidance. They trust us. How could they do that if we behave indifferently to them and their loved one and the struggle that lies before them? If I could recommend the impossible, I would advise all healthcare workers to spend time in these two areas. It's telling of who cares and who does not care about other human beings. Those who are capable of compassion and connecting become clear. Unfortunately, that is unrealistic, and we can't use this as tool to weed out indifference. That would be undignified and careless of us. It does raise the question however, how to breed caring and compassion in our staff.

What is the point of all this? Why did I write this? It's not because I'm trying to bash our hospitals. The truth is we have a number of hospitals that are doing very well in the way they care for patients. I love what we do in our health systems. Being part of a hospital and witnessing the miracles performed is beyond exhilarating and rewarding. Transplanting hearts and lungs that give human beings a second chance at life is miraculous. I feel that we need reminders that those miracles are living, breathing human beings. Our focus has been misplaced. There is a piece of caring we're forgetting: Humanity, returning human connection, respect and dignity to our practices.

I shared the stories I did because they were so demonstrative of how we've forgotten that these people, our patients, are human. They are someone's mother, father, brother or sister. They may be someone's daughter or son. The entire world around us has contributed to the indifference that has engulfed much of our staff. There are a number of policies and programs that organizations are trying to use successfully, but if the members of your staff are not living the culture you are creating it will not work. How do you find staff who live it? You find the 1 in 4 employees who are constantly trying to sink the ship. If they need to go, they go. You find the ones who care about their work and want to be fulfilled by delivering more than customer service. The ones who want to deliver an excellent human experience.

Everything we do in this life is a human experience, whether you think of it that way or not. If you focus on delivering human experiences, the patient experience that dictates patient satisfaction scores will sky rocket. Your staff will finally love their work again. Call me a dreamer. Call me old-fashioned, but how did the world survive before all this? What made the world go round before technology and industrial revolution? The people of the world had to count on one another. They had to trust each other. They had to care about each other. They had to connect in all the ways we're struggling to connect these days. It was the only way they survived.

When we talk about culture statements, I give you the same example. What was the culture back in the days of old? The culture was one of community. The people in a community, came together to help his neighbor cultivate the land and reap the harvest. The same goes for our culture when caring for patients. We must have a culture of community. To come together and lay the ground work, cultivate the land in order to see the success, reap the harvest and enjoy the fruit of our labors. One cannot change it on their own with just one voice. Many can come together and join voices to speak up and be the change the healthcare world has been waiting for. As we cultivate our new clinical professionals, we can teach them to live the culture of caring, of community. When we help one, we help many. Have you or anyone you've seen sat down with a patient, held their hand, and just let them know you care? I've seen what it can do, and it can be a simple act, but the result can be miraculous. It's human, it's trust, and it's care. Is that appropriate for all patients? No. Are there other ways to connect with patients? Yes, many. When we work in an environment that cultivates caring and humanity and we learn how to reinforce it every day, our employees begin to live it. Again, is there a cost? There is always a cost. The better question is what are the benefits?

Susan C. Dewey

"You can't depend on your eyes when your imagination is out of focus."

~Mark Twain

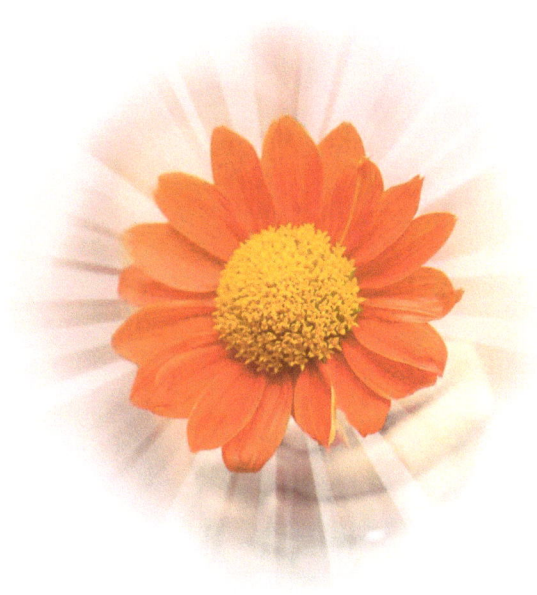

Chapter 14

SHIFTING THE PARADIGM

When we focus only on the numbers, we miss the most important component to healthcare—the care. Think of it this way: If patients could answer these two questions on the Patient Satisfaction Survey with consistent 10's, consider what would have to happen to the rest of the scores with little effort. The first question, "How would you rate us on a scale of 1 to 10?" The second, "How likely is it you would recommend us to a friend?" First of all, could they score us a 10 if we didn't deliver a true human experience? I don't believe so. Could they consistently score us a 10 if we gave them a nosocomial infection? Probably not. Could they score us a 10 if we operated on the wrong limb? I don't believe so. Would a patient score us a 10 if we consistently failed to do trach care and they suffered over 3 ½ hours of trach and wound care, when a doctor wouldn't take the time to remove sutures? Of course not. Would the frail woman on the BiPAP, who didn't get to eat breakfast, rate you a 10 on these two questions? I doubt it.

Until we're working in a way that decreases these types of incidents, you will not be consistently scored a 10 on these two questions, which can be used to drive the rest of your patient satisfaction scores. We cannot change how Medicare, Medicaid and our insurance companies function or fail to function properly.

We cannot change the federal law or mandates put in place. What we can do is realize those things may never change. So what can we do to make our systems work better under the current legislation? What do we need to do to take The Affordable Care Act and make it work in our favor? For starters, consider that many problems are swept under the rug and not discussed or addressed. How does an administrator or director know there's a problem when we keep covering it up with falsified charting? Or making sure our staff keeps quiet thru intimidation?

There was an occasion that I was assigned an 18-bed ICU and assigned to 2 other floors. Because my ICU patients were in need of critical care and ongoing interventions, I could not get to the other 2 floors to administer treatments. I called my team leader to tell him I would need help getting them done. He was responsible as our team leader to manage the situation. I noticed at the end of the day, he had not charted or removed the treatments from the medication record on the computer. I was assigned to them so I handled the charting. I charted "treatment not given" because he had told me that he couldn't get to a couple of them because they were eating breakfast. We are required to chart *why* it wasn't given. I charted that I was not available to give the treatment, because I wasn't. I was up to my eye balls in ICU duties.

The next day I was approached by a manager and told that I had to go back and change my charting because we are not allowed to chart that we were unavailable. I was told to either change the charting to "patient unavailable or patient refused". I informed the manager that I had not seen the patient and was unable to speak for my team leader and why he didn't give the treatments. If they wanted it changed, it was up to the team leader to change it. My charting was accurate. This is what I mean by covering problems up. How does anyone know we have dangerous staffing issues if we falsify charting to accommodate the reports our directors run? Our director has to explain those reports and does not want anyone charting that we are not available because it reflects poorly on them and our department. Considering the staffing problems we face in respiratory and nursing, I find this approach counterproductive.

Many nurses and care givers want to speak up, and want to see changes but are discouraged and afraid to do so.

We are about to enter a new Medicare territory called community based care. What does that mean? It means making sure people in our community are seeking and receiving preventative care and as a result, preventing hospital admissions or re-admissions. Hospital readmissions are an area of patient satisfaction scores hospitals focus on but fail to recognize the tools to reduce these re-admissions. The best way to reduce re-admissions and begin executing community based programs is to follow our patients even after discharge. A number of our patients get confused easily. When they get home and don't understand the instructions or medications, they end up back in our emergency departments. With my own children, I have gone home believing I understand the instructions and medications, only to end up having a million questions. What if they aren't improving or the medicine is causing bad side effects? Follow up calls help in this situation.

You may be asking yourself, am I more interested in patient satisfaction scores, or patient care? I am discussing both, because it's impossible to ignore the relationship between the two. Working on one improves the other. If I could say something I believe many other caregivers would like to say, it would be this: Your best tool, and most valuable resource in your arsenal to fight indifference and improve your patients experience, it's your front line staff and your patients.

The concept most misused when applied to patient care is customer service and service excellence. It's customer service to an extent. But let me ask you this, how good is the customer service you receive when you are the customer these days? What if everyone, including businesses, returned to using a human touch—knowing customers names, patient's names, their likes and dislikes, looking them in the eye and smiling when they are speaking, acknowledging their presence, sympathizing with them, holding their hand or reaching out to embrace them if they need a hug? Studies have shown that human touch decreases stress and anxiety levels. They release oxytocin, which make us feel good. Whether being applied to business or healthcare, treating people like human beings benefits all of humanity.

You may be thinking this is crazy. These ideas won't work in our hospital. Why not? Why couldn't it? It might cost too much? Well, if you take the great things we already do well in healthcare, such as performing miracles, and the many medical advances in the past 50 years, why is it crazy to think there is a better way to care for the people those miracles and advances were designed to save? How would we accomplish this? Could it mean rethinking and redesigning our processes for caring? It could mean rethinking the job duties in each role. An overlapping of skills or duties that makes our teams more collaborative. More training for physicians and holding them to a new standard which requires them to treat others with the same respect they wish to be treated?

When we look at the issues from a different perspective, we're better equipped to find solutions. That's innovation, and that's what paves the road for new, advanced ideas and techniques. Where would we be today without fresh, new, innovative thinking? Look where technology and the world have advanced as a result of those who were able to think outside the box. In healthcare, thinking outside the box may also mean, thinking inside our hearts and recognizing that those on the receiving end of our services, are human beings.

We may not have the ability to change legislation which dictates Medicare, Medicaid and insurance, but we can find a way to treat our patients with the dignity and respect we all appreciate ourselves, and as a result improve their patient experience and outcomes. The definition of insanity is doing the same thing over and over again, only to find the same results. We keep doing the same things that were done 50 years ago, that are no longer working. Yet, we're expecting a new result, better care and higher patient satisfaction scores. Doesn't it just make sense? How do you wish to be treated, especially when you are sick? Do we enjoy being ignored? Do any of us like to feel like we're a burden to someone who is caring for us? Do any of us appreciate our privacy and dignity? We all prefer to be treated like human beings, but for that to happen it has to begin somewhere, with one person. Could that person be you?

The next time the phrase pops in your head, "I'm just a nurse," or "Just a Respiratory Therapist," "Just a tech or PCA," remember you have the ability to make a difference in people's lives. You are the one who decides whether that happens or not. Try saying it again and remove the word "Just." Go back to standing up for your patients and their care; be the difference, be a leader. It's time we realize the important role we play in the care of our patients. We may not be doctors—so what? That doesn't make us less important. The doctor's work is useless without us to make it happen. We heal the sick every day; we're at the bedside. We deliver the medications, manage the care, make the calls, place the orders, carry out the treatment plans that the doctors initiate. They do not outrank us, we do not outrank them or each other if we're part of a cohesive team; all members of the care team share equal responsibility and equal importance. We're each one person, who can only do so much. One cannot do it all on their own, we count on each other, as our patients count on us. When patient care returns to the forefront, our roles will be united, forming a seamless team, who can deliver human experiences and thoughtful, intentional patient care rather than indifference.

All it takes is one, to say "I care, even if no one else does."

Susan C. Dewey

REFERENCES

Studer, Q. (2003). Hardwiring excellence: Purpose worthwhile work making a difference. Gulf Breeze, FL: Fire Starter Pub. ISBN: 9780974998602

RATIOS: Assessment. (n.d.). Retrieved September 23, 2015.

http://www.nationalnursesunited.org/pages/ratios-assessment

David Feinberg youtube Quality Improvement and Healthcare Reform: Patient Experience with David Feinberg (Visit: http://www.uctv.tv/) Published on May 24, 2012

Healthcare Expert, Author, & CEO of Studer Group. Quint Studer, CEO & Founder of Studer Group, Published on July 10, 2013

Keynote Speaker: Quint Studer • Presented by SpeakInc • Innovation and Sustainable Change

ABOUT THE AUTHOR

Susan Dewey is a Motivational Speaker, Patient Advocate and Consultant aiming to revolutionize the patient experience and medical outcomes by putting the "care" back in healthcare. She has 12 years of experience in health care in both the Midwest and Southeastern United States.

Susan is currently an RRT-Registered Respiratory Therapist. Each day, she uses her signature, "flower power," — a nod to the pink-flowered hair clip she wears daily — to connect with her patients and brighten their most difficult days.

Her passion for providing caregivers a voice and making a difference in patients' lives is heavily shaped not only by her day-to-day experience in the field, but by her family's battles with cancer, end of life decisions, and with those entrusted with their care.

www.ingramcontent.com/pod-product-compliance
Lightning Source LLC
Chambersburg PA
CBHW040904180526
45159CB00010BA/2924